PLANT BASED DIET COOKBOOK 2021

50 Easy and affordable recipes that beginners and advanced can cook in easy steps. Quick & Easy meals for busy people to lose weight fast.

Ursa Males

TABLE OF CONTENTS

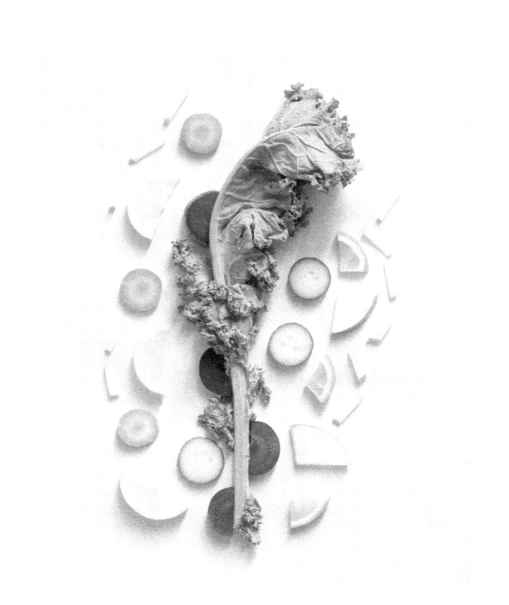

BREAKFAST

1. <u>Dairy-Free Coconut Yogurt</u>

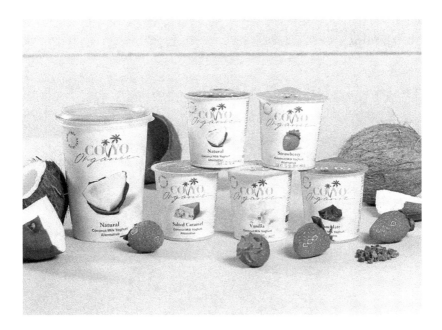

Preparation time: 5 minutes

Cooking time: 0 minutes

Servings: 2

Ingredients:

- 1 can coconut milk
- 4 vegan probiotic capsules

Directions:

1. Shake coconut milk with a whole tube. Remove the plastic capsules and mix in. Cut a 12-inch cheesecloth until stirred. Freeze or eat immediately.

Nutrition: Calories: 219 Fat: 10.1g Carbohydrates:1.5g Protein: 7.9g

2. <u>Vegan Green Avocado Smoothie</u>

Preparation time: 5 minutes

Cooking time: 0 minutes

Servings: 2

Ingredients:

- 1 banana
- 1 cup of water
- 1/2 avocado
- 1/2 lemon juice
- 1/2 cup coconut yogurt

Directions:

1. Blend all fixings until smooth. Serve.

Nutrition: Calories: 299 Fat: 1.1g Carbohydrates: 1.5g Protein: 7.9g

3. <u>Sun-Butter Baked Oatmeal Cups</u>

Preparation time: 10 minutes

Cooking time: 25 minutes

Servings: 12 cups

Ingredients:

- 1/4 cup coconut sugar
- 11/2 rolled oats
- 2 tablespoon chia seeds
- 1/4 teaspoon salt
- 1 teaspoon cinnamon
- 1/2 cup non-dairy milk
- 1/2 cup Sun-Butter
- 1/2 cup apple sauce

Directions:

1. Preheat oven to 350°F. Mix all fixings and blend well. Add in muffins and put extra toppings. Bake 25 minutes, or until golden brown.

Nutrition: Calories: 129 Fat: 1.1g Carbohydrates: 1.5g Protein: 4.9g

4. <u>Chocolate Peanut Butter Shake</u>

Preparation time: 5 minutes

Cooking time: 0 minutes

Servings: 2 servings

Ingredients:

- 2 bananas
- 3 Tablespoons peanut butter
- 1 cup almond milk
- 3 Tablespoons cacao powder

Directions:

1. Combine fixings in a blender until smooth.

Nutrition: Calories: 149 Fat: 1.1g Carbohydrates: 1.5g Protein: 7.9g

5. <u>The Husband Protein Smoothie</u>

Preparation Time: 3 minutes

Cooking time: 0 minute

Servings: 1

Ingredients:

- 1/4 cup rolled oats
- 1 cup wild blueberries, frozen
- 1-inch fresh ginger, peeled and diced
- 1 cup strawberries, frozen
- 3 tablespoon hulled hemp seeds
- 2 cups baby spinach
- 2 tablespoon almond butter
- 2 tablespoon maple syrup
- 1 1/4 cups of water

Directions:

1. Add all fixings into the blender and blend for a minute or until it looks smooth.

Nutrition: Calories: 680 Carbs: 84g Proteins: 21g Fat: 36g

6. <u>Caramel Chia Seed Pudding</u>

Preparation Time: 10 minutes

Cooking time: 0 minutes

Servings: 4

Ingredients:

- 1 cup date caramel
- 2 1/8 oz chia seeds
- 2 tablespoon maple syrup
- 1 cup of coconut milk
- 1 teaspoon vanilla extract
- 1/4 cup water
- A pinch of salt

Directions:

1. In a blender, add coconut milk, chia seeds, salt, vanilla, maple syrup, and water. Properly blend this mixture until smooth.
2. Place the blended mixture into a sealed container and refrigerate for about 2 hours or overnight.
3. Get a jar and add the date caramel before the refrigerated coconut milk mixture. Do this for about 4 layers in one jar.

Nutrition: Calories: 316 Carbs: 50g Protein: 4.4g Fats: 13g

7. __Banana Waffles__

Preparation Time: 5 minutes

Cooking time: 5 minutes

Servings: 6

Ingredients:

- 1/4 teaspoon ground nutmeg
- 1 cup cashew milk, unsweetened
- 1 teaspoon ground cinnamon
- 2 1/2 tablespoon cashew butter
- 1/4 teaspoon baking soda
- 1 peeled medium banana
- 1 tablespoon baking powder
- 7 oz all-purpose flour
- 2 tablespoon sugar

Directions:

1. In a blender, add all the Ingredients: on the list, cashew milk, and baking soda first. Blend for a minute until smooth.
2. In a waffle maker, use a spoon to transfer the mixture and cook the batter over medium-high heat. Your machine might not tell you when they are ready.

3. Take them off when you can no longer see steam.

Nutrition: Calories: 200 Carbs: 35g Protein: 4g Fat: 5g

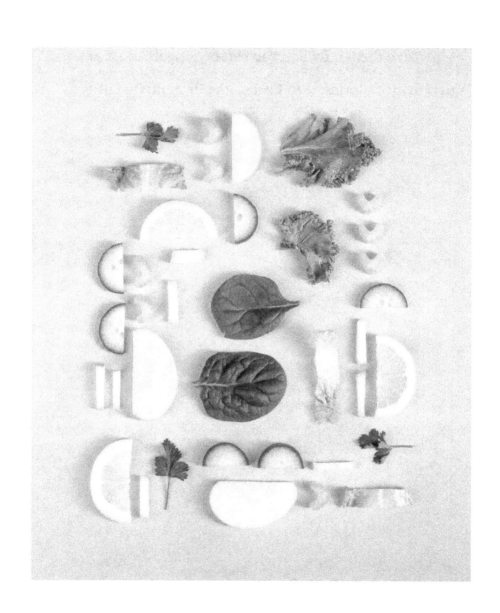

LUNCH

8. Special Jambalaya

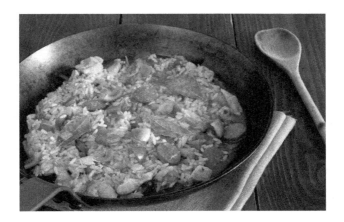

Preparation time: 10 minutes

Cooking time: 6 hours

Servings: 4

Ingredients:

- 6 ounces soy chorizo, chopped
- 1 and ½ cups celery ribs, chopped
- 1 cup okra
- 1 green bell pepper, chopped
- 16 ounces canned tomatoes and green chilies, chopped
- 2 garlic cloves, minced
- ½ teaspoon paprika
- 1 and ½ cups veggie stock

- a pinch of cayenne pepper
- black pepper to the taste
- a pinch of salt
- 3 cups already cooked wild rice for serving

Directions:

1. Warm-up a pan over medium-high heat, put soy chorizo, stir, brown for a few minutes and transfer to your slow cooker.
2. Also, add celery, bell pepper, okra, tomatoes and chilies, garlic, paprika, salt, pepper, and cayenne to your slow cooker.
3. Stir everything, add the veggie stock, cover the slow cooker, and cook on low for 6 hours. Divide rice between plates, top each serving with your vegan jambalaya and serve hot. Enjoy!

Nutrition: Calories 150 Fat 3g Carbs 15g Protein 9g

9. <u>Chinese Tofu and Veggies</u>

Preparation time: 10 minutes

Cooking time: 4 hours

Servings: 4

Ingredients:

- 14 ounces extra-firm tofu, pressed & cut into medium triangles
- cooking spray
- 2 teaspoons ginger, grated
- 1 yellow onion, chopped
- 3 garlic cloves, minced
- 8 ounces tomato sauce
- ¼ cup hoisin sauce
- ¼ teaspoon coconut aminos
- 2 tablespoons of rice wine vinegar
- 1 tablespoon soy sauce
- 1 tablespoon spicy mustard
- ¼ teaspoon red pepper, crushed
- 2 teaspoons molasses
- 2 tablespoons water
- a pinch of black pepper
- 3 broccoli stalks

- 1 green bell pepper, cut into squares
- 2 zucchinis, cubed

Directions:

1. Warm-up a pan over medium-high heat, add tofu pieces, brown them for a few minutes and transfer to your slow cooker.
2. Heat the pan again over medium-high heat, add ginger, onion, garlic, and tomato sauce, stir, sauté for a few minutes and transfer to your slow cooker as well.
3. Add hoisin sauce, aminos, vinegar, soy sauce, mustard, red pepper, molasses, water, and black pepper, stir gently, cover, and cook on high for 3 hours.
4. Add zucchinis, bell pepper, and broccoli, cover, and cook on high for 1 more hour. Divide between plates and serve right away.

Nutrition: Calories 300 Fat 4g Carbs 14g Protein 13g

10. Corn Chowder

Preparation time: 10 minutes

Cooking time: 8 hours and 30 minutes

Servings: 6

Ingredients:

- 2 cups yellow onion, chopped
- 2 tablespoons olive oil
- 1 red bell pepper, chopped
- 1 pound gold potatoes, cubed
- 1 teaspoon cumin, ground
- 4 cups corn kernels
- 4 cups veggie stock
- 1 cup almond milk
- a pinch of salt
- a pinch of cayenne pepper
- ½ teaspoon smoked paprika
- chopped scallions for serving

Directions:

1. Warm-up a pan with the oil over medium heat, add onion, stir and sauté for 5 minutes and then transfer to your slow cooker.

2. Add bell pepper, 1 cup corn, potatoes, paprika, cumin, salt, and cayenne, stir, cover and cook on low for 8 hours.
3. Blend this using an immersion blender and then mix with almond milk and the rest of the corn.
4. Stir chowder, cover, and cook on low for 30 minutes more. Ladle into bowls and serve with chopped scallions on top.

Nutrition: Calories 200 Fat 4g Carbs 13g Protein 16g

11. **<u>Black Eyed Peas Stew</u>**

Preparation time: 10 minutes

Cooking time: 4 hours

Servings: 8

Ingredients:

- 3 celery stalks, chopped
- 2 carrots, sliced
- 1 yellow onion, chopped
- 1 sweet potato, cubed
- 1 green bell pepper, chopped
- 3 cups black-eyed peas, soaked for 8 hours, and drained
- 1 cup tomato puree
- 4 cups veggie stock
- A pinch of salt
- Black pepper to the taste
- 1 chipotle chili, minced
- 1 teaspoon ancho chili powder
- 1 teaspoons sage, dried and crumbled
- 2 teaspoons cumin, ground
- Chopped coriander for serving

Directions:

1. Put celery in your slow cooker. Add carrots, onion, potato, bell pepper, black-eyed peas, tomato puree, salt, pepper, chili powder, sage, chili, cumin, and stock.
2. Stir, cover, and cook on High within 4 hours. Stir stew again, divide into bowls and serve with chopped coriander on top. Enjoy!

Nutrition: Calories 200 Fat 4g Carbs 9gProtein 16g

12. **White Bean Cassoulet**

Preparation time: 10 minutes

Cooking time: 6 hours

Servings: 4

Ingredients:

- 2 celery stalks, chopped
- 3 leeks, sliced
- 4 garlic cloves, minced
- 2 carrots, chopped
- 2 cups veggie stock
- 15 ounces canned tomatoes, chopped
- 1 bay leaf
- 1 tablespoon Italian seasoning
- 30 ounces canned white beans, drained

For the breadcrumbs:

- Zest from 1 lemon, grated
- 1 garlic clove, minced
- 2 tablespoons olive oil
- 1 cup vegan bread crumbs
- ¼ Cup parsley, chopped

Directions:

1. Heat a pan with a splash of the veggie stock over medium heat, add celery and leeks, stir and cook for 2 minutes. Add carrots and garlic, stir and cook for 1 minute more.
2. Add this to your slow cooker and mix with stock, tomatoes, bay leaf, Italian seasoning, and beans. Stir, cover, and cook on low within 6 hours.
3. Meanwhile, heat a pan with the oil over medium-high heat, add bread crumbs, lemon zest, 1 garlic clove, and parsley, stir, and toast for a couple of minutes.
4. Divide your white beans mix into bowls, sprinkle bread crumbs mix on top and serve. Enjoy!

Nutrition: Calories 223 Fat 3g Carbs 10g Protein 7g

13.   Light Jackfruit Dish

Preparation time: 10 minutes

Cooking time: 6 hours

Servings: 4

Ingredients:

- 40 ounces green jackfruit in brine, drained
- ½ cup agave nectar
- ½ cup gluten-free tamari sauce
- ¼ cup soy sauce
- 1 cup white wine
- 2 tablespoons ginger, grated
- 8 garlic cloves, minced
- 1 pear, cored and chopped
- 1 yellow onion, chopped
- ½ cup water
- 4 tablespoons sesame oil

Directions:

1. Put jackfruit in your slow cooker. Add agave nectar, tamari sauce, soy sauce, wine, ginger, garlic, pear, onion, water, and oil.
2. Stir well, cover, and cook on low within 6 hours. Divide jackfruit mix into bowls and serve. Enjoy!

Nutrition: Calories 160 Fat 4g Carbs 10g Protein 3g

14. **Veggie Curry**

Preparation time: 10 minutes

Cooking time: 4 hours

Servings: 4

Ingredients:

- 1 tablespoon ginger, grated
- 14 ounces canned coconut milk
- cooking spray
- 16 ounces firm tofu, pressed and cubed
- 1 cup veggie stock
- ¼ cup green curry paste
- ½ teaspoon turmeric
- 1 tablespoon coconut sugar
- 1 yellow onion, chopped
- 1 and ½ cup red bell pepper, chopped
- a pinch of salt
- ¾ cup peas
- 1 eggplant, chopped

Directions:

1. Put the coconut milk in your slow cooker. Add ginger, stock, curry paste, turmeric, sugar, onion, bell pepper, salt, peas, and eggplant pieces, stir, cover and cook on high for 4 hours.

2. Meanwhile, spray a pan with cooking spray and heat up over medium-high heat. Add tofu pieces and brown them for a few minutes on each side.

3. Divide tofu into bowls, add slowly cooked curry mix on top, and serve. Enjoy!

Nutrition: Calories 200 Fat 4g Carbs 10g Protein 9g

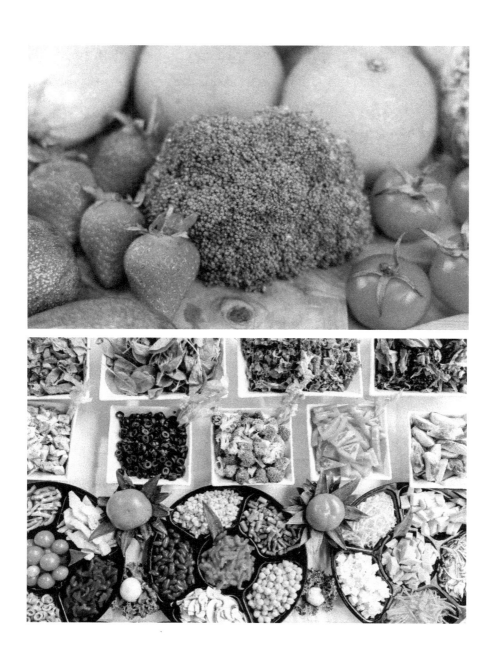

DINNER

15. The Medi-Wrap

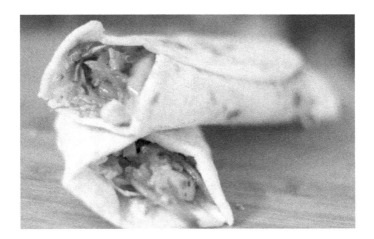

Preparation time: 5 minutes

Cooking time: 0 minutes

Servings: 6

Ingredients:

- ¼ cup crispy chickpeas
- ¼ cup cherry tomatoes halved
- Handful baby spinach
- 2 romaine lettuce leaves, for wrapping
- 2 tablespoons lemon juice, fresh
- ¼ cup hummus
- 2 tablespoons kalamata olives, quartered

Directions:

1. Take a bowl and mix in all ingredients except hummus and lettuce leaves, stir well. Put hummus over lettuce leaves, top with the chickpea mixture. Wrap them up and serve. Enjoy!

Nutrition: Calories: 55 Fat: 0g Carbohydrates: 12g Protein: 3g

16. Nectarine and Quinoa

Preparation time: 15 minutes

Cooking time: 1 hour & 15 minutes

Servings: 6

Ingredients:

- ½ cup kale, chopped
- 1/3 cup pumpkin seeds, roasted
- 3 tablespoons lemon vinaigrette
- 1/3 cup scallions, sliced thin
- 1 cup quinoa, cooked and room temperature
- 2 nectarines, chopped into ½ inch wedges
- ½ cup white cabbage, shredded

Directions:

1. Take a bowl and add all listed ingredients, stir well. Serve and enjoy!

Nutrition: Calories: 400 Fat: 18g Carbohydrates: 52g Protein: 11g

17. Grilled Sprouts and Balsamic Glaze

Preparation time: 15 minutes

Cooking time: 30 minutes

Servings: 2

Ingredients:

- ½ pound Brussels sprouts, trimmed and halved
- Fresh cracked black pepper
- 1 tablespoon olive oil
- Sunflower seeds to taste
- 2 teaspoons balsamic glaze
- 2 wooden skewers

Directions:

1. Take wooden skewers and place them on a large piece of foil. Place sprouts on the skewers and with drizzle oil, sprinkle sunflower seeds and pepper. Cover skewers with foil.
2. Pre-heat your grill to low and place skewers (with foil) in the grill. Grill for 30 minutes, making sure to turn after every 5-6 minutes. Once done, uncover and drizzle balsamic glaze on top.

Nutrition: Calories: 440 Fat: 27g Carbohydrates: 33g Protein: 26g

18. Green Creamy Cabbage

Preparation time: 15 minutes

Cooking time: 10 minutes

Servings: 4

Ingredients:

- 2 ounces almond butter
- 1 and ½ pounds green cabbage, shredded
- 1 and ¼ cups of coconut cream
- Sunflower seeds and pepper to taste
- 8 tablespoons fresh parsley, chopped

Directions:

1. Put almond butter in a skillet over medium heat, and let it melt. Add cabbage and sauté until browns.
2. Stir in cream and turn down the heat to low. Let it simmer. Season with sunflower seeds and pepper. Garnish with parsley and serve. Enjoy!

Nutrition: Calories: 432 Fat: 42g Carbohydrates: 8g Protein: 4g

19. Rice Mushroom Risotto

Preparation time: 15 minutes

Cooking time: 15 minutes

Servings: 4

Ingredients:

- 4 and ½ cups cauliflower, riced
- 3 tablespoons coconut oil
- 1-pound Portobello mushrooms, thinly sliced
- 1-pound white mushrooms, thinly sliced
- 2 shallots, diced
- ¼ cup organic vegetable broth
- Sunflower seeds and pepper to taste
- 3 tablespoons chives, chopped
- 4 tablespoons almond butter
- ½ cup kite ricotta/cashew cheese, grated

Directions:

1. Pulse cauliflower florets using a food processor until rice. Take a large saucepan and heat up 2 tablespoons of oil over a medium-high flame.

2. Put mushrooms and sauté for 3 minutes until mushrooms are tender. Clear saucepan of mushrooms and liquid and keep them to one side.

3. Add the last tablespoon of oil to the skillet. Toss shallots and cook for 60 seconds. Add cauliflower rice, stir for 2 minutes until coated with oil.

4. Add broth to riced cauliflower and stir for 5 minutes. Remove pot from heat and mix in mushrooms and liquid.

5. Add chives, almond butter, and ricotta/cheese. Season with sunflower seeds and pepper. Serve and enjoy!

Nutrition: Calories: 438 Fat: 17g Carbohydrates: 15g Protein: 12g

20. __Almond and Blistered Beans__

Preparation time: 15 minutes

Cooking time: 20 minutes

Servings: 4

Ingredients:

- 1-pound of fresh green beans ends trimmed
- 1 and ½ tablespoons olive oil
- ¼ teaspoon sunflower seeds
- 1 and ½ tablespoons fresh dill, minced
- Juice of 1 lemon
- ¼ cup crushed almonds
- Extra sunflower seeds as needed

Directions:

1. Preheat your oven to 400degree Fahrenheit. Add in the green beans with your olive oil and also with sunflower seeds.

2. Then spread them in one single layer on a large-sized sheet pan. Roast it up for 10 minutes and stir it nicely, then roast for another 8-10 minutes

3. Remove it from the oven and keep stirring in the lemon juice alongside the dill. Top it with crushed almonds and some sunflower seeds and serve

Nutrition: Calories: 347 Fat: 16g Carbohydrates: 6g Protein: 45g

21. **Tomato Platter**

Preparation time: 2-3 hours & 15 minutes

Cooking time: 0 minutes

Servings: 8

Ingredients:

- 1/3 cup olive oil
- 1 teaspoon sunflower seeds
- 2 tablespoons onion, chopped
- ¼ teaspoon pepper
- ½ a garlic, minced
- 1 tablespoon fresh parsley, minced
- 3 large fresh tomatoes, sliced
- 1 teaspoon dried basil
- ¼ cup red wine vinegar

Directions:

1. Take a shallow dish and arrange tomatoes in the dish. Add the rest of the ingredients in a mason jar, cover the jar and shake it well. Pour mix over tomato slices. Let it chill for 2-3 hours. Serve!

Nutrition: Calories: 350 Fat: 28g Carbohydrates: 10g Protein: 14g

22.   Garbanzo and Spinach Beans

Preparation time: 15 minutes

Cooking time: 0 minutes

Servings: 4

Ingredients:

- 1 tablespoon olive oil
- ½ onion, diced
- 10 ounces spinach, chopped
- 12 ounces garbanzo beans
- ½ teaspoon cumin

Directions:

1. Take a skillet and add olive oil, let it warm over medium-low heat. Add onions, garbanzo and cook for 5 minutes. Stir in spinach, cumin, garbanzo beans and season with sunflower seeds
2. Use a spoon to smash gently. Cook thoroughly until heated, enjoy!

Nutrition: Calories: 90 Fat: 4g Carbohydrates:11g Protein:4g

SNACKS

23. Cinnamon-Lime Sunflower Seeds

Preparation time: 5 minutes

Cooking time: 5 minutes

Servings: 8

Ingredients:

- 1 cup sunflower seeds
- 1 tablespoon sugar, maple syrup, or Simple Syrup
- Pinch salt
- 1 tablespoon freshly squeezed lime juice
- 1 to 2 teaspoons ground cinnamon or pumpkin pie spice

Directions:

1. Put the sunflower seeds in a large skillet, and cook over medium heat, tossing continuously, for 3 to 5 minutes, until lightly browned.

2. Add the sugar and salt, and keep tossing the seeds. Remove from the heat, and add the lime juice and cinnamon, tossing quickly to coat while the juice sizzles.

Nutrition: Calories: 169Protein: 5gFat: 14gCarbohydrates: 8g

24. **Bruschetta**

Preparation time: 15 minutes

Cooking time: 5 minutes

Servings: 4

Ingredients:

- 1 tomato, finely diced
- 1 tablespoon chopped onion or scallion
- Salt
- ½ baguette, sliced, or 2 bread slices
- 1 tablespoon olive oil
- Freshly ground black pepper

Directions:

1. Toss the tomato, onion, and a pinch of salt in a small bowl. Transfer to a strainer, and let drain in the sink or over a bowl for a few minutes while you prep the bread. Toast the bread lightly.
2. Return the drained tomato mixture to the bowl, drizzle with the olive oil, and season to taste with pepper.
3. If using full slices of bread, cut each in half. Scoop the tomato batter on top of the toasts right before serving.

Nutrition: Calories: 70Protein: 2gFat: 4gCarbohydrates: 7g

25. **Classic Hummus & Veggies**

Preparation time: 15 minutes

Cooking time: 0 minutes

Servings: 6

Ingredients:

- 1 (15-ounce) can chickpeas, drained and rinsed
- 1 garlic clove, minced
- ¼ cup freshly squeezed lemon juice, or to taste
- ¼ cup tahini
- 2 tablespoons olive oil
- ¼ to ½ teaspoon salt, or to taste
- 2 to 3 tablespoons water
- Crudités, such as carrot sticks, cucumber slices, or cherry tomatoes, or crackers and pita bread, for serving

Directions:

1. Combine the chickpeas, garlic, lemon juice, tahini, olive oil, and salt in a food processor. Purée until fully combined, stopping to scrape down the sides of the bowl, as needed.

2. Put the water, 1 tablespoon at a time, until you get a smooth and creamy consistency. Transfer to a bowl and serve with your choice of dippers.

Nutrition: Calories: 222Protein: 7gFat: 11gCarbohydrates: 26g

26. **Parsley & White Bean Dip**

Preparation time: 15 minutes

Cooking time: 0 minutes

Servings: 6

Ingredients:

- 1 (15-ounce) can white beans, drained & rinsed
- ¼ cup fresh parsley
- 1 scallion, white & light green parts only, chopped
- 2 tablespoons olive oil, or 1 tablespoon tahini plus 2 tablespoons water
- 1 tablespoon apple cider vinegar
- 1 tablespoon nutritional yeast
- 1 teaspoon dried herbs
- ¼ teaspoon salt, plus ¼ teaspoon more if needed

Directions:

1. In a food processor or small blender, combine the white beans, parsley, scallion, olive oil, vinegar, nutritional yeast, dried herbs, and ¼ teaspoon salt.
2. Purée until fully combined, stopping to scrape down the sides as needed.

3. Taste after puréeing, and add the remaining salt, if desired. Transfer to a bowl and serve.

Nutrition: Calories: 104Protein: 5gFat: 5gCarbohydrates: 11g

27. 5-Layer Dip

Preparation time: 15 minutes

Cooking time: 0 minutes

Servings: 6

Ingredients:

- 1½ cups Refried Beans
- 1 cup Loaded Guacamole
- 1 cup Sour Cream
- ½ cup chopped pitted olives
- 2 or 3 tomatoes, diced
- ¼ cup salsa
- ½ cup grated vegan cheese (optional)
- Tortilla chips, for serving

Directions:

1. Spread the refried beans in an 8-inch baking dish, followed by the guacamole, sour cream, and olives.
2. In a small bowl, stir together the tomatoes and salsa, and spread this mixture over the top of the dip.

3. Sprinkle on the cheese (if using), and serve with tortilla chips for dipping.

Nutrition: Calories: 329Protein: 8gFat: 17gCarbohydrates: 38g

VEGETABLES

28. Minted Peas

Preparation Time: 5 minutes

Cooking Time: 5 minutes

Serving: 4

Ingredient:

- 1 tablespoon olive oil
- 4 cups peas, fresh or frozen (not canned)
- ½ teaspoon sea salt
- Freshly ground black pepper
- 3 tablespoons chopped fresh mint

Direction:

1. In a large sauté pan, cook olive oil over medium-high heat until hot.
2. Add the peas and cook, about 5 minutes. Remove the pan from heat.

3. Stir in the salt, season with pepper, and stir in the mint. Serve hot.

Nutrition: 90 Calories 5g Fiber 8g Protein

29. **Sweet and Spicy Brussels Sprout Hash**

Preparation Time: 10 minutes

Cooking Time: 15 minutes

Serving: 4

Ingredient:

- 3 tablespoons olive oil
- 2 shallots, thinly sliced
- 1½ pounds Brussel sprouts
- 3 tablespoons apple cider vinegar
- 1 tablespoon pure maple syrup
- ½ teaspoon sriracha sauce (or to taste)
- Sea salt
- Freshly ground black pepper

Direction

1. In pan, cook olive oil over medium-high heat until it shimmers.
2. Mix the shallots and Brussels sprouts and cook, stirring frequently, until the -vegetables soften and begin to turn golden brown, about 10 minutes.
3. Stir in the vinegar, using a spoon to scrape any browned bits from the pan's bottom. Stir in the maple syrup and Sriracha.

4. Simmer, stirring frequently, until the liquid reduces, 3 to 5 minutes. Season and serve immediately.

Nutrition: 97 Calories 4g Fiber 7g Protein

SALAD

30. **Italian Veggie Salad**

Preparation Time: 10 minutes

Cooking Time: 0 minutes

Servings: 8

Ingredients:

For salad:

- 1 cup fresh baby carrots, quartered lengthwise
- 1 celery rib, sliced
- 3 large mushrooms, thinly sliced
- 1 cup cauliflower florets, bite sized, blanched
- 1 cup broccoli florets, blanched
- 1 cup thinly sliced radish
- 4-5 ounces' hearts of romaine salad mix to serve

For dressing:

- ½ package Italian salad dressing mix
- 3 tablespoons white vinegar
- 3 tablespoons water
- 3 tablespoons olive oil
- 3-4 pepperoncino, chopped

Directions:

To make salad:

1. Add all the ingredients of the salad except hearts of romaine to a bowl and toss.

To make dressing:

2. Add all the ingredients of the dressing in a small bowl. Whisk well.
3. Pour dressing over salad and toss well. Refrigerate for a couple of hours.
4. Place romaine in a large bowl. Place the chilled salad over it and serve.

Nutrition: Calories 84Total Fat 6.7gSaturated Fat 1.2g

Cholesterol 3mgSodium 212mgTotal Carbohydrate 5gDietary Fiber 1.4gTotal Sugars 1.6gProtein 2gVitamin D 31mcg

Calcium 27mgIron 1mgPotassium 193mg

GRAINS

31. Pecan-Maple Granola

Preparation Time: 5 minutes

Cooking Time: 50 minutes

Servings: 4

Ingredients:

- 1½ cups rolled oats
- ¼ cup maple syrup (optional)
- ¼ cup pecan pieces
- 1 teaspoon vanilla extract
- ½ teaspoon ground cinnamon

Directions:

1. Preheat the oven to 300°F (150°C). Line a baking sheet with parchment paper.
2. In a large bowl, stir together all the ingredients until the oats and pecan pieces are completely coated.
3. Spread the mixture on the baking sheet in an even layer. Bake in the oven for 20 minutes, stirring once halfway through cooking.

4. Remove from the oven and allow to cool on the countertop for 30 minutes before serving.

Nutrition: calories: 221fat: 17.2gcarbs: 5.1gprotein: 4.9g fiber: 3.8g

32. Bean and Summer Squash Sauté

Preparation Time: 10 minutes

Cooking Time: 15 to 16 minutes

Servings: 4

Ingredients:

- 1 medium red onion, peeled and thinly sliced
- 4 yellow squash, cut into ½-inch rounds
- 4 medium zucchinis, cut into ½-inch rounds
- 1 (15-ounce / 425-g) can navy beans, drained and rinsed
- 2 cups corn kernels
- Zest of 2 lemons
- 1 cup finely chopped basil
- Salt, to taste (optional)
- Freshly ground black pepper, to taste

Directions:

1. Place the onion in a large saucepan and sauté over medium heat for 7 to 8 minutes. Add water 1 to 2 tablespoons at a time to keep the onion from sticking to the pan.
2. Add the squash, zucchini, beans, and corn and cook for about 8 minutes, or until the squash is softened.

3. Remove from the heat. Stir in the lemon zest and basil. Season with salt (if desired) and pepper.
4. Serve hot.

Nutrition: calories: 298fat: 2.2g carbs: 60.4gprotein: 17.2gfiber: 13.6g

LEGUMES

33. Creamed Green Pea Salad

Preparation Time: 10 minutes

Cooking Time: 10 minutes

Servings: 4

Ingredients:

- 2 (14.5 ounce) cans green peas, drained
- 1/2 cup vegan mayonnaise
- 1 teaspoon Dijon mustard
- 2 tablespoons scallions, chopped
- 2 pickles, chopped
- 1/2 cup marinated mushrooms, chopped and drained
- 1/2 teaspoon garlic, minced
- Sea salt and ground black pepper, to taste

Directions

1. Place all the ingredients in a salad bowl. Gently stir to combine.
2. Place the salad in your refrigerator until ready to serve.

3. Bon appétit!

Nutrition: Calories: 154; Fat: 6.7g; Carbs: 17.3g; Protein: 6.9g

34. **Middle Eastern Za'atar Hummus**

Preparation Time: 10 minutes

Cooking Time: 10 minutes

Servings: 4

Ingredients:

- 10 ounces' chickpeas, boiled and drained
- 1/4 cup tahini
- 2 tablespoons extra-virgin olive oil
- 2 tablespoons sun-dried tomatoes, chopped
- 1 lemon, freshly squeezed
- 2 garlic cloves, minced
- Kosher salt and ground black pepper, to taste
- 1/2 teaspoon smoked paprika
- 1 teaspoon Za'atar

Directions

1. Blitz all the ingredients in your food processor until creamy and uniform.
2. Place in your refrigerator until ready to serve.
3. Bon appétit!

Nutrition: Calories: 140; Fat: 8.5g; Carbs: 12.4g; Protein: 4

BREAD & PIZZA

35. Keto Mug Bread

Preparation time: 2 minutes

Cooking time: 2 minutes

Servings: 1

Ingredients:

- 1/3 cup Almond Flour
- 1/2 teaspoon Baking Powder
- 1/4 teaspoon Salt
- 1 Whole Egg
- 1 tablespoon Melted Butter

Directions:

1. Mix all ingredients in a microwave-safe mug.
2. Microwave for 90 seconds.
3. Cool for 2 minutes.

Nutrition: Calories 416 Carbohydrates 8 g Fats 37 g Protein 15 g

36. **<u>Keto Blender Buns</u>**

Preparation time: 5 minutes

Cooking time: 25 minutes

Servings: 6

Ingredients:

- 4 Whole Eggs
- 1/4 cup Melted Butter
- 1/2 teaspoon Salt
- 1/2 cup Almond Flour
- 1 teaspoon Italian Spice Mix

Directions:

1. Preheat oven to 425-degree F.
2. Pulse all ingredients in a blender.
3. Divide batter into a 6-hole muffin tin.
4. Bake for 25 minutes.

Nutrition: Calories 200 Carbohydrates 2 g Fats 18 g Protein 8 g

SOUP AND STEW

37. Zucchini Soup

Preparation Time: 10 minutes

Cooking Time: 15 minutes

Servings: 8

Ingredients:

- 2 ½ lbs zucchini, peeled and sliced
- 1/3 cup basil leaves
- 4 cups vegetable stock
- 4 garlic cloves, chopped
- 2 tbsp olive oil
- 1 medium onion, diced
- Pepper
- Salt

Directions:

1. Heat olive oil in a pan over medium-low heat.
2. Add zucchini and onion and sauté until softened. Add garlic and sauté for a minute.
3. Add vegetable stock and simmer for 15 minutes.

4. Remove from heat. Stir in basil and puree the soup using a blender until smooth and creamy. Season with pepper and salt.
5. Stir well and serve.

Nutrition: Calories: 434 kcal Fat: 35gCarbs: 27gProtein: 6.7g

38. Creamy Celery Soup

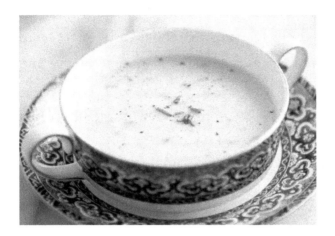

Preparation Time: 20 minutes

Cooking Time: 20 minutes

Servings: 4

Ingredients:

- 6 cups celery
- ½ tsp dill
- 2 cups water
- 1 cup coconut milk
- 1 onion, chopped
- Pinch of salt

Directions:

1. Add all ingredients into the electric pot and stir well.
2. Cover electric pot with the lid and select soup setting.
3. Release pressure using a quick release method than open the lid.
4. Puree the soup using an immersion blender until smooth and creamy.
5. Stir well and serve warm.

Nutrition: Calories: 159kcalFat: 8.4gCarbs: 19.8g Proteins: 4.6g

SAUCES, DRESSINGS & DIP

39. Chimichurri

Preparation time: 10 minutes

Cooking time: 5 minutes

Servings: 8

Ingredients:

- 1/2 yellow bell pepper, deseeded and finely chopped
- 1 green chili pepper, deseeded and finely chopped
- Juice and zest of 1 lemon
- 1 cup olive oil
- 1/2 cup parsley, chopped
- 2 garlic cloves, grated
- Salt and pepper to taste

Directions:

1. Add all **Ingredients:** to a large mixing bowl. Can be mixed with by hand or with an immersion blender. Mix until desired consistency is achieved.

2. Can be served over burgers, sandwiches, salads and more. Can be stored in the refrigerator for up to 5 days or for longer in the freezer.

Nutrition: Total fat: 25.3g Sodium: 3mg Fiber: 2g

40. Keto Vegan Raw Cashew Cheese Sauce

Preparation time: 5 minutes

Cooking time: 5 minutes

Servings: 6

Ingredients:

- 1 cup raw cashews, soaked in water for at least 3 hours before making recipe
- 2 tablespoons olive oil
- 2 tablespoon nutritional yeast
- 1/4 teaspoon garlic powder
- 2 tablespoons fresh lemon juice
- 1/2 cup water
- Salt to taste

Directions:

1. To prepare cashews before making the sauce, boil 2 cups of water turn off heat and add cashews. This can be allowed to soak overnight. Rinse and strained cashews. Discard water.

2. Add all **Ingredients:** to a food processor and blend until a smooth consistency is achieved. Can be used to make pizzas, over roasted veggies, in lasagna, as a dip and more.

Nutrition: Total fat: 15.5g Sodium: 34mg Total carbohydrates: 9.23g Protein: 5.1g

APPETIZER

41. Homemade Hummus

Preparation Time: 15 minutes

Cooking Time: 0 minutes

Servings: 8

Ingredients:

- 30 ounces (2 cans) garbanzo beans
- 1/3 cup chickpea liquid
- ½ cup tahini
- ¼ cup olive oil
- 2 lemons, juiced
- 2 teaspoons garlic, minced
- ½ teaspoon salt

Directions:

1. Add all ingredients to a blender. Blend until smooth for about 30 seconds.
2. Transfer to an airtight container and sprinkle with additional seasonings or olive oil if desired.

Nutrition: 330 calories Fat 17 g Protein 12 g Carbs 35 g

42. **Spinach and Artichoke Dip**

Preparation Time: 20 minutes

Cooking Time: 10 minutes

Servings: 10

Ingredients:

- 1 tablespoon olive oil
- 2 teaspoons garlic, minced
- 12 ounces marinated artichoke hearts
- 4 cups baby spinach, roughly chopped
- ¼ cup vegan mayonnaise
- 8 ounces vegan cream cheese
- ½ teaspoon onion powder
- ½ teaspoon salt

Directions:

3. Preheat the oven to 400°F. Add olive oil, garlic, artichoke hearts, and spinach to skillet. Sauté for about 3 minutes to soften the vegetables.
4. Add cream cheese, mayo, and spices. Mix until well incorporated. Add the mixture to an oven-safe baking dish. Broil for 5 minutes.

5. Remove from the oven and serve warm with crackers or chips.
6. This recipe is great to bring to social events.

Nutrition: Calories 75Fat 6 g Protein 3 g Carbs 5 g

SMOOTHIES AND JUICES

43. Strawberry and Chocolate Milkshake

Preparation time: 5 minutes

Cooking time: 0 minute

Servings: 2

Ingredients:

- 2 cups frozen strawberries
- 3 tablespoons cocoa powder
- 1 scoop protein powder
- 2 tablespoons maple syrup
- 1 teaspoon vanilla extract, unsweetened
- 2 cups almond milk, unsweetened

Directions:

1. Place all the ingredients in the order in a food processor or blender and then pulse for 2 to 3 minutes at high speed until smooth.

2. Pour the smoothie into two glasses and then serve.

Nutrition: Calories: 199 Cal Fat: 4.1 g Carbs: 40.5 g Protein:3.7 g Fiber: 5.5 g

44. **Trope-Kale Breeze**

Preparation Time: 5 minutes

Cooking Time: 0 minute

Servings: 3 to 4 cups

Ingredients:

- 1 cup chopped pineapple (frozen or fresh)
- 1 cup chopped mango (frozen or fresh)
- ½ to 1 cup chopped kale
- ½ avocado
- ½ cup coconut milk
- 1 cup water, or coconut water
- 1 teaspoon matcha green tea powder (optional)

Directions:

1. Purée everything in a blender until smooth, adding more water (or coconut milk) if needed.

Nutrition: Calories: 566Total fat: 36gCarbs: 66gFiber: 12gProtein: 8g

DESSERTS

45. Almond and Chocolate Chip Bars

Preparation time: 45 minutes

Cooking time: 0 minutes

Servings: 10

Ingredients:

- 1/2 cup almond butter
- 1/4 cup coconut oil, melted
- 1/4 cup agave syrup
- 1 teaspoon vanilla extract
- 1/4 teaspoon sea salt
- 1/4 teaspoon grated nutmeg
- 1/2 teaspoon ground cinnamon
- 2 cups almond flour
- 1/4 cup flaxseed meal
- 1 cup vegan chocolate, cut into chunks
- 1 1/3 cups almonds, ground
- 2 tablespoons cacao powder
- 1/4 cup agave syrup

Directions:

1. In a mixing bowl, thoroughly combine the almond butter, coconut oil, 1/4 cup of agave syrup, vanilla, salt, nutmeg and cinnamon.

2. Gradually stir in the almond flour and flaxseed meal and stir to combine. Add in the chocolate chunks and stir again.

3. In a small mixing bowl, combine the almonds, cacao powder and agave syrup. Now, spread the ganache onto the cake. Freeze for about 30 minutes, cut into bars and serve well chilled. Enjoy!

Nutrition: Calories: 295Fat: 17gCarbs: 35.2gProtein: 1.7g

46. **Almond Butter Cookies**

Preparation time: 45 minutes

Cooking time: 12 minutes

Servings: 10

Ingredients:

- 3/4 cup all-purpose flour
- 1/2 teaspoon baking soda
- 1/4 teaspoon kosher salt
- 1 flax egg
- 1/4 cup coconut oil
- 2 tablespoons almond milk
- 1/2 cup brown sugar
- 1/2 cup almond butter
- 1/2 teaspoon ground cinnamon
- 1/2 teaspoon vanilla

Directions:

1. Mix the flour, baking soda plus salt in a mixing bowl. In another bowl, combine the flax egg, coconut oil, almond milk, sugar, almond butter, cinnamon and vanilla.
2. Stir the wet batter into the dry fixings and stir until well combined.

3. Place the batter in your refrigerator for about 30 minutes. Shape the batter into small cookies and arrange them on a parchment-lined cookie pan.

4. Bake at 350 degrees F within 12 minutes in a preheated oven. Move the pan to your wire rack to cool at room temperature. Bon appétit!

Nutrition: Calories: 197Fat: 15.8gCarbs: 12.5gProtein: 2.1g

47. **Peanut Butter Oatmeal Bars**

Preparation time: 15 minutes

Cooking time: 20 minutes

Servings: 20

Ingredients:

- 1 cup vegan butter
- 3/4 cup coconut sugar
- 2 tablespoons applesauce
- 1 ¾ cups old-fashioned oats
- 1 teaspoon baking soda
- A pinch of sea salt
- A pinch of grated nutmeg
- 1 teaspoon pure vanilla extract
- 1 cup oat flour
- 1 cup all-purpose flour

Directions:

1. Warm your oven to 350 degrees F. In a mixing bowl, thoroughly combine the dry ingredients. In another bowl, combine the wet ingredients.
2. Then, stir the wet mixture into the dry ingredients; mix to combine well.

3. Spread the batter mixture in a parchment-lined square baking pan. Bake within 20 minutes. Enjoy!

Nutrition: Calories: 161Fat: 10.3gCarbs: 17.5gProtein: 2.9g

48. Vanilla Halvah Fudge

Preparation time: 1 hour & 15 minutes

Cooking time: 0 minutes

Servings: 16

Ingredients:

- 1/2 cup cocoa butter
- 1/2 cup tahini
- 8 dates, pitted
- 1/4 teaspoon ground cloves
- A pinch of grated nutmeg
- A pinch coarse salt
- 1 teaspoon vanilla extract

Directions:

1. Prepare a square baking pan lined using parchment paper.
2. Mix the ingredients until everything is well incorporated.
3. Scrape the batter into the parchment-lined pan.
4. Place in your freezer until ready to serve.

5. Bon appétit!

Nutrition: Calories: 106Fat: 9.8gCarbs: 4.5gProtein: 1.4g

49. <u>**Raw Chocolate Mango Pie**</u>

Preparation time: 3 hours & 15 minutes

Cooking time: 0 minutes

Servings: 16

Ingredients:

Avocado layer:

- 3 ripe avocados, pitted and peeled
- A pinch of sea salt
- A pinch of ground anise
- 1/2 teaspoon vanilla paste
- 2 tablespoons coconut milk
- 5 tablespoons agave syrup
- 1/3 cup cocoa powder

Crema layer:

- 1/3 cup almond butter
- 1/2 cup coconut cream
- 1 medium mango, peeled
- 1/2 coconut flakes
- 2 tablespoons agave syrup

Directions:

1. In your food processor, blend the avocado layer until smooth and uniform; reserve. Then, blend the other layer in a separate bowl. Spoon the layers in a lightly oiled baking pan.

2. Transfer the cake to your freezer for about 3 hours. Store in your freezer. Bon appétit!

Nutrition: Calories: 196Fat: 16.8gCarbs: 14.1gProtein: 1.8g

50. **Keto Cheesecake**

Preparation time: 30 minutes

Cooking time: 1 hour & 5 minutes

Servings: 6

Ingredients:

For the crust:

- 2 cups almond flour
- 1/3 cup butter, melted
- 2 tablespoons granulated erythritol
- 1 teaspoon vanilla extract
- For the filling:
- 32 ounces cream cheese, at room temperature
- 1 cup powdered erythritol
- 3 large organic eggs
- 1 tablespoon freshly squeezed lemon juice
- 1 teaspoon vanilla extract
- For the topping:
- 1 cup diced strawberries
- ½ tablespoon freshly squeezed lemon juice
- ¼ cup granulated erythritol

Directions:

1. For the crust, warm your oven to 350°F. Spray a 9-inch springform pan with cooking spray. In a medium bowl, stir together the almond flour, butter, erythritol, and vanilla until a crumbly dough form.
2. Press the crust into the bottom of the prepared pan and bake for around 9 minutes. Remove and allow to cool.
3. For the filling, use a handheld electric mixer to mix together the cream cheese and powdered erythritol in a separate bowl until blended.
4. Add the eggs and continue to beat until well combined. Put the lemon juice and vanilla and beat for another minute. Pour the filling into the cooled pie crust. Bake for 45 minutes, then set on a rack to cool.
5. For the topping, stir the topping ingredients in a small saucepan over medium-low heat, and simmer, stirring occasionally, for 15 to 20 minutes.
6. Remove from the heat and allow to cool to room temperature.
7. Then place the topping in a blender or food processor and pulse 5 to 7 times.